## ABOUT THE AUTHOR

Zachariah Evans is the byname of a journalist and broadcaster who became well-known as an entrepreneur. Evans founded one of the first coffee bars, the first chain of steak house restaurants, as well as one of Britain's most enduring nightclubs.

He discovered his cure for sleeplessness during a crisis that wrecked his sleep and nearly ruined his life.

He has written cook books, a novel and, most recently, with G. Theresa Wintour, "Guide To Village Riches", for those wishing to get away from the city and enjoy life and business in the countryside, where he himself now lives with his second wife.

# SLEEPLESSNESS CURED:
# THE DRUG-FREE, QUICK and PROVEN WAY

## Zachariah Evans

**Saturday
Richmond
Publishers**

# SLEEPLESSNESS CURED:  THE DRUG-FREE, QUICK AND PROVEN WAY

Copyright (c) SATURDAY RICHMOND PUBLISHERS 1991
All rights reserved.

Copies of this publication have been lodged with
The Agent for The Copyright Libraries, 100 Euston St,
London NW1 2HO;
and The Legal Deposit Office, British Library,
Boston Spa, Wetherby, W. Yorks LS23 7BW

Published by Saturday Richmond Publishers
for The Insomnia & Snoring Cure Group,
Northavon, BS12 3PR

First impression October 1991
Second impression February 1992

**British Library Cataloguing
in Publication Data**
Evans, Zachariah
   Sleeplessness Cured: the drug-free,
quick and proven way.

Bibliography
Index
I. Title
616.8498

ISBN 1-872804-04-7

Typeset, printed and bound in Great Britain by
The Guernsey Press Co. Ltd, Guernsey, Channel Islands.

# INTRODUCTION

I found myself involved in a particularly bitter divorce and custody law suit some years ago; under the intense pressure I changed from an energetic go-getter into a withdrawn and resentful wreck.

As the conflict dragged on I realised that if I was to survive I would need much resolution and, above all, I would have to keep a cool head. The problem was that rational thought was increasingly difficult because the restful slumber that I'd enjoyed all my life was becoming a memory – I was sleeping very badly. However, amidst all the fire and brimstone I finally homed in on a simple therapy and, as a result, I was able to rediscover drug-free, quality sleep and thereby reach calmer waters.

Since my discovery I have proved the success of my sleep formula by sharing it with many friends and acquaintances, so a booklet aimed at helping a wider audience seemed called for. If you are sleeping badly, remember that I understand the problem and in the following pages you will find the solution. This drug-free cure for sleeplessness has only ever done good, never harm to anyone; perhaps more than can be said for the sleeping pills and tranquillisers often prescribed for the condition.

PRESENTATION: In Section One are the essential methods that will give you quality sleep, and details of interesting but optional sleep aids that may make going to bed more appealing. Section Two sketches current scientific sleep research. Section Three examines matters that negatively affect sleep; eg, sleeping pills and snoring. Section Four contains a short look at some oddities of sleep. In Section Five you will find details of books and other information sources mentioned in the text; also sources of help and a few tips for dealing with some other problems not mentioned in the text but which typically keep an awful lot of people miserable and awake at night.

# CONTENTS

# SECTION ONE

---

## CHAPTER 1:   HOW TO GET REGULAR, QUALITY SLEEP

As we spend about a third of our lives in sleep it is clearly important that this time is spent enjoyably and usefully, in refreshing ourselves, so that we can live happy and normal lives. However, science believes that 50% of the UK population suffer from sleep problems at sometime or the other. Often these problems will take the form of worrying and sleep-destructive thoughts intruding to prevent the onset of sleep or proving so powerful that frequent awakenings occur during the night.

### QUALITY SLEEP:   YOUR BUTTRESS FOR LIFE
Whilst for some the bad sleep patch may pass, for many others the sleeplessness will continue (and perhaps be made worse by taking sleeping pills). For these sufferers my drug-free sleep formula will give you back quality sleep and, importantly, will buttress your sleep against any situation you may meet in the future. The formula does not take long to learn and once you have mastered the simple and pleasant routine outlined in the next few pages you will be able to sleep well whatever life decides to throw at you. Let me also stress that my sleep formula can be learned at any age; a toddler old enough to converse can learn it, as can those of advanced years.

### MY SLEEP FORMULA — THE BASIC STEPS
- Rise each morning at a regular, convenient hour.
- By doing so regain control of your day and mental ease.
- Pay attention to a few commonsense ideas on diet.
- Construct a relaxed pre-bed routine.
- Use a hobby to construct your sleep-thought.
- Experiment to find the sleep hours you really need.

You will not be familiar with my expression "sleep-thought". As this is the most important part of your sleeplessness cure, I will, of course, be explaining it later in detail. Meanwhile, just consider this: It is impossible to think steadily about more than one thing at a time. If you like, give yourself a few seconds and test that statement now. For example, try and think in a concentrated way about what you're actually going to cook for this evening's dinner and at the same time try and think about exactly which teams you are going to mark with an X to win you a million on the weekend's football pools.

You will find that you can maintain one *or* the other thought process; not both at once. For those who are sleeping poorly, one thought at a time will provide the vital missing link in the chain of events that ends in sleeping soundly.

Before we get to that point, however, we need to look at the beginning of the chain, the start of your day.

## LATE START PROBLEMS

For example, if, because of tiredness, you fail to make an on-time start and constantly arrive for work at 10 or 11 o'clock when you should be starting at 9, you are not going to have a very good day, nor a job or business for very long, because the start of your day is disorganised. Equally, if you put yourself under constant tension to make your day-start deadline it's evident that something is wrong with your waking-up and early-morning routines.

Your excuse will be that you are sleeping badly and that fact makes a desirable early-rise habit difficult, if not impossible, to achieve. Perhaps true – until now.

## BE AN EARLY BIRD

What is to be done is not, as you might think, to leave your waking-up problem until after we have you sleeping soundly, but the reverse. By putting into effect what follows you are taking the first, very positive action towards curing your poor sleep, as will become clear in a moment. Here's how it works:–

Having carefully worked out your *ideal* daily time to get up (probably much earlier than at present), at an hour that will give you comfortable time to rise leisurely, dress as you would wish, breakfast nourishingly, have a look at the paper, cope easily with the traffic snarls and get you to the desk or job with time in hand – having decided on that time, when it arrives each morning – *get up*.

Do I hear an agonised groan? Perhaps, but we are not going to be deterred by the probability that you have previously struggled with and failed to solve this problem of early rising. Very likely you have been relying on an alarm clock; excellent machines, but far too easy to switch off, allowing you to roll over and go back to sleep, guilty conscience and all. Enough of all that failure! There is a method that guarantees you will get up at the correct time, whether you want to or not:–

## YOUR BODY AS ALARM CLOCK
You will train your bladder to be your alarm clock.

We each have a personal bladder cycle. A few days' study of your own will tell you when and under what liquid-intake circumstances you pass water. The bladder holds up to one pint of urine and most people produce around three pints per day. Most of us urinate before the bladder is full, i.e. between four and six times per day. As your doctor will confirm, you can train your bladder by adjusting the timing and amount of your liquid intake so that it will be possible in a relatively short time to then "match" your morning urination with the time you want to get up.

(There is another reason why training your bladder is an essential exercise. When you have got your sleep working successfully, as you will, you do not want it to be interrupted in the middle of the night by having to get up to relieve yourself. Remember, just as the mind cannot cope with more than one thought at a time, neither can you stay asleep if you're bursting.)

## YOUR MIND AS ALARM CLOCK
In addition to using your body as a clock you can also use your mental "clock" to get you up at the required time in the morning. According to sleep scientists, we somehow "monitor" the passing of time whilst we sleep. By habitually telling yourself at bedtime how many hours later you want to get up the next morning you are programming yourself to awaken at that hour. Practice this and you will quickly find that your mental and body alarm clocks will combine together to have you out of bed and into your early-morning routine.

## YOUR DOG WILL HELP, TOO
We can marshal your body and mind to effect early rising; perhaps there is a further method or back-up that can be used? If you are fortunate enough to have a dog he can be enrolled to further motivate you and make early rising more pleasurable: Put your alarm clock nearby your pet's sleep place and, when the alarm goes off, train him to stir and make a bit of a fuss at your new getting-up time. How do you get him to do this? Easy, really; few dogs can resist the treat of a morning walk; not to mention that the fresh air helps clear the cobwebs in a sleepy head.

You have probably been in the habit of snatching an extra hour or so in bed at the weekends. You may not care for what follows but, to start with, I ask you to get up at the same time every day; yes, even on Saturdays and Sundays. After you have complete mastery of your early-rise routine then by all means sleep in at the weekends if you wish, but a variety of getting-up times to begin with will confuse your inner rhythms and make the habit of regular, early rising more difficult to acquire.

It won't have escaped you that by waking up at the same early time each morning you will, if you have slept badly beforehand, feel pretty sleepy during the day. Hard going though this will be, try not to let this disturb you unduly because this tiredness is both going to be short-lived and in a very real way is going to help you rapidly towards a sleeplessness cure, as I will show you.

## REGAINING CONTROL OF THE GAME

Let's go forward on the basis that you are regularly getting up at your "right" time. The first and most important prize that you've won is the recapture of a large measure of control over your life. No longer the rush, tension, anger and frustration of constantly racing the clock, of mumbled apologies for lateness, of shame. However sleepy you may be, *you* are ahead of the game in terms of time.

Invaluably, you will have also boosted your confidence in the knowledge and belief that you have laid the foundation for a solution to your sleeplessness.

## UNDERLYING TROUBLES

Another window of opportunity also opens: With that extra, precious time that is now yours you have the opportunity to think about other matters. Could it be that there are things that have been troubling you? However imperfectly we think when we are tired, it is still important to at least acknowledge the fact if a problem exists. In due course you will need to deal with your problem and in Chapter Seven I offer some other insights into how you can meet and beat troublesome barriers to sleep.

I should emphasise here that, even though you do have one or several problems that trouble you so much that they have been affecting your sleep, we will still get you to sleep well. Nevertheless, we are looking for the best quality sleep; nagging worries do affect this.

Apart from addressing underlying problems, please also monitor how you handle your ordinary day-time activities because this will have an effect on how easily you get off to sleep at night. With less rush you will find it easier to avoid getting anxious and uptight, resentful and angry – powerful and negative feelings that frequently persist until bedtime and, if they do, will impede efforts to get off to sleep. It is also useful to try and remember that each new dawn heralds the first day of the rest of your life. You will best serve yourself and others around you if you are relaxed and effective, so getting the best possible from each of these days; try consciously to enjoy life.

## APPROACHING BEDTIME

What I want us to do now is to consider the preparations for the night's sleep.

Let us proceed on the platform of your having had your less-hassled day. You're home from the office or have finished the day's chores and are looking forward to some well-earned relaxation.

If you fear that I'm going to nanny you into changing any of those pleasures, relax; eg, experts reckon that moderate drinking in the evening can be beneficial, so you will probably continue to enjoy your usual few pints in the pub, or home with a bottle of wine, some TV, a book or chatting with family or friends. In reasonable moderation, whatever pleases you, enjoy. All I do ask is that you leave at least two hours between your evening meal and going to bed. The primary digestion process is not helpful to sound sleep.

## CHECK OUT YOUR DIET

Whilst on the question of food and drink you might ask yourself whether your chronic tiredness is not being made even worse by a food or drink allergy. Also consider your diet balance; eg, tests carried out as long ago as the Sixties found that magnesium and potassium supplements had a startling and positive effect on chronically tired volunteers, in some cases enabling them to feel much livelier and more refreshed on fewer than their usual number of hours sleep. If you suspect that allergy and/or diet investigations might help you then see your GP or holistic therapist for further advice. See Section Five for books that may be useful.

## PRE-BED ROUTINE

Please give regard to your immediate pre-bed routine. Ensure that this is methodical and leisurely as far as possible, doing much the same things at much the same time each night. The object is to get the beginning of this routine to signal the brain that you are getting ready for sleep.

Once you are in the bedroom there may be something else to think about: You are your own guv'nor and if you enjoy your sex at bedtime, so be it. However, sex can be even more stimulating than perhaps you think. After it you may fall quickly into a very deep, short sleep but then awake to find getting back to sleep difficult. On the other hand if, unhappily, the sex wasn't great your frustration may impede you getting off. Perhaps sex earlier in the day or evening would be best for you. Consider.

Now, to bed:

## INTRUDERS NOT WELCOMED

Let us visualise that you have completed your leisurely pre-bed routine and are tucked up comfortably in bed. Remember that you have satisfied yourself that your mind can only handle one thought at a time. You will not, therefore, lie tense, wondering whether or not you're going to be able to get off to sleep or, indeed, mentally entertaining *any* other problem – you will replace negative thought by a positive thought that you *do* want. You will

11

then hold *that* thought, your sleep-thought, in your mind. Quite shortly you will be asleep.

To further explain: Although we do not yet fully understand the mind, we all know that "choosing" and "willing" are two of its functions. So, faced with the choice of either fretting and staying awake or thinking about something that will get you to sleep, what are you going to do? Choose the sleep-thought and "will" out the thought you *know* is keeping you awake, of course.

## THE PLEASURE PRINCIPLE

This process is helped by consciously harnessing what unconsciously makes you put off thinking about your problems during the day: Rather than think about something unpleasant or distressing you use instead what is called "the pleasure principle"; you put the painful aside and think about something more pleasant. Which gives us the final clue: My sleep formula works because you obtain relief from the mental anguish of a negative thought and obtain *pleasure* from the sleep-thought with which you will replace it.

It remains therefore for you to decide what this positive, pleasant thought will be *about*.

## FINDING YOUR SLEEP-THOUGHT

Well, now, this is surely not going to be difficult. However miserable you are there will be at least one subject that you find enjoyable to think about. Whilst I cannot know what it is, it will exist and we can give it a name: your hobby; a favourite subject or occupation that is not your main business.

The best example I have of the hobby as sanity- and sleep-saver is my own. I should mention that, perhaps like you, I have the sort of mind that "locks" onto a project or problem. This is good during the day, but, when in crisis some years ago my mind suddenly started to lock onto the problem when I was trying to get to sleep, this resulted in a most harmful and continual disruption of my sleep.

## HEALING THE SELF-INFLICTED WOUND

My salvation emerged with the twin insights that (a) my sleeplessness was a self-inflicted wound; it was not my opponents who were forcing negative bedtime thoughts into my head – it was me who was allowing them access. What followed from this was (b) that I needed to drive out the bad thoughts and replace them with pleasing ones. But where could I look for pleasant thoughts in the middle of a crisis?

The answer proved to be my passion for lawn tennis in general and the Wimbledon Lawn Tennis Singles Championships in particular. I set about learning the dates my Wimbledon heroes and heroines had won this Championship, who they had played in the final and the score. Within a few days (for I was desperate to test my theory) I had learned my list★ and I began my experiment. Frankly, for the first few nights I struggled somewhat, with unwelcome thoughts occasionally but stubbornly breaking through, but on or about the fifth night I managed to silently recite my list without any intrusive thoughts being able to muscle in and disrupt the onset of sleep. I slept the sleep of the dead. When I awoke it was as if to a new life. (Maybe it was no coincidence that very soon afterwards my crisis began to subside!)

My hobby, the Wimbledon Championships, began in 1877. Since that date there have been over 100 meetings. It is rare that I am not slumbering soundly long before I mentally reach the present-day champions; I am usually asleep within five minutes of going to bed. A little pleasant learning about your own hobby and you will get exactly the same reward.

★See precise details of my hobby list on page 17.

**THE "GROUND RULES"**
In Chapter Two you will find out all about the hobby/sleep-thought formula but now it is necessary to tell you about the "ground rules" which will ensure that you get utmost benefit.

Should you be in any doubt that bedtime is the wrong time to entertain problems then consider this: What we know about the brain tells us that it is still by far the most powerful "machine" in the universe. It is also ceaselessly active, which is fine during the day when you can "will" it to coherence, a disaster at bedtime when the brain can pump out uncontrolled and random half-thoughts that mingle restlessly with your tiredness and leave you fretful and sleepless. Daytime is for mental challenges and problems, bedtime is for controlled sleep-thoughts and for sleep.

The purpose in mentioning this is to underline the need for discretion in your choice of replacement, positive sleep-thought. For example, if you are a chess player please do *not* pose yourself new chess problems; you will be awake until the small hours and beyond whilst the grey matter gleefully chases up hill and down dale finding half-baked "solutions" that won't stand up to the cold light of day, anyway. By all means in your mind *replay* games, but don't invent and try to play games as yet *un*played. Please.

In short, the experience you are buying says that your hobby sleep-thought should beneficially concentrate on what *has* happened (the historical), the *non-speculative*.

Therefore, silently recite to yourself your factual list, firmly willing aside any other negative thoughts that try to intrude and very soon your pleasant thoughts will bond with your tiredness to ensure good slumber.

## SLEEP THROUGH PLEASURE

Once the simple logic of the formula is accepted you will be pleasantly surprised at how very easily you can master this new use of your hobby. Because you really enjoy the subject of your recitation you will find that each night your sleep-thought works more easily. Within a short while you will be self-trained to go to sleep virtually at will. Your will. No drugs.

Earlier on I asked you not to let your daytime tiredness bother you unduly. The reason is that my sleep formula embraces the necessity to be *really* tired when you go to bed. The combination of this healthy tiredness and your sleep-thought ensures quality sleep.

## SHARING YOUR BED

Once you have trained yourself to quickly and easily get off to sleep and stay asleep you will get maximum benefit by then finding out the right number of hours of sleep for *you*. Here's how this is done and, as you will see, there are perhaps several factors to consider:-

Earlier I mentioned sex. Also involving your partner is another potentially ticklish matter: If your bed is shared you could find that your partner's activity during the night (a person can make as many as 300 movements during sleep) is affecting your already troubled sleep. Might there be a case for separate beds?

Separate beds may also feature for another reason: You are unique so you will have your own sleep requirements. How many hours per night you need (bearing in mind your fixed early-rise time each morning) will be found by experimenting with the times at which you go to bed at night. Your ideal retirement time may well be different to your partner's; with this as a possibility, separate beds would ensure that the earlier-to-bed is not disturbed by the arrival of the later-to-bed.

Shared double beds and the same bedtime no doubt work for many couples; for others, they don't.

## THE RIGHT HOURS FOR YOU

There is no *average,* "ideal" number of hours of sleep. Whilst history does not record anyone ever having survived for long without any sleep at all, there are some remarkable cases of people positively thriving on as little as two or three hours sleep a night. At the other extreme, nine hours or more is considered essential by many. There is also another factor: As you will see from Chapter Four, some scientists wonder if we should be taking all of our sleep in one chunk. Eg, supposing you find that you get off to sleep nicely but regularly wake up in the middle of the night. It could well be that your sleep pattern is calling for you to stop fretting about getting off to sleep again and, instead, requires you to get up and work or do some reading for an hour or so before then going back to bed and a quick and effortless return to sleep.

**The only yardstick that matters is what works for you; what number of hours' quality sleep you need to awake refreshed, have a 100% day and get into bed at night feeling healthily tired and ready to drop off and sleep your required hours.**

Unrealistic sleep expectations, ie tossing and turning with worry about the number of hours convention makes you think you *ought* to be sleeping will only damage your sleep. If your real need is to sleep more or less than what you've been brought up to believe is necessary, then don't be surprised — and let no one talk you out of getting that special number of hours in *your* way. You alone are the judge.

**TO SUMMARISE**
1.  Quality sleep is essential for a contented life and is the best defence against troubled times.
2.  You begin winning control of your sleep and your life by rising early, regardless of resulting tiredness, which is an important component in the eventual cure.
3.  Early rising gives you time to work unhassled and also to consider underlying troubles. Mental ease means getting to sleep quicker and more easily.
4.  Moderate relaxation habits need not be changed but diet should be considered and at least two hours allowed for digestion before retiring.
5.  A pre-bed routine is essential.
6.  You might consider if sex at bedtime is the right time for you.
7.  Successful sleeping is based upon the fact of being able to think about only one thing at a time. Your hobby list is used as the basis for your sleep-thought which will keep negative thoughts at bay. Observe the "ground rules".
8.  Separate beds may need consideration.
9.  Experiment is necessary to find the number of hours sleep that are right for you.


# CHAPTER 2:  MORE ON HOBBY LISTS
## & HOW TO USE THEM

For passing interest, the word "hobby" comes to us via the wickerwork "hobby-horse" on which actors perform amusing antics as part of the Morris dances. Their object? Of course, to please.

**GUARANTEEING QUALITY SLEEP**
It is not putting it too high to say that, by rediscovering your senses of pleasure and satisfaction in some hobby or interest and putting them to use in the way I propose, you are guaranteeing yourself quality sleep.

What that hobby, that pleasure, is for you I cannot tell, but that doesn't matter at all; I only suggest that you do stick to the ground rules I have mentioned: Concentrate on what *has happened* in your hobby, not what *might* have happened. To begin with, I recommend you concentrate on **lists with dates;** these have the virtue of being most easily remembered, which will help to lead you forward to the next item; you know that if you miss out an item your list will be incomplete. This will make you concentrate that little bit more.

## AN IMPORTANT "TRICK"
Perhaps the single most important "trick" to ensure the success of my sleep formula is to *always begin* by recalling the *identical* facts; eg, as you will see with my own hobby sleep–thought, I always start with the year, the name of the winner, who he beat and the score. Taking that one important step further, I have found that reciting just "1877" is enough to "trigger" the command my brain is awaiting that *I have decided to go to sleep.* My brain is trained now to obey that command and I am seldom if ever troubled by the brain wanting to bull–doze in other unwanted thoughts; it learned long ago that I will reject them. With "1877" recited, almost immediately I begin to feel consciousness slipping away.

As the symmetry and harmony of what you are recalling gives you greater and greater pleasure and contentment, you will find that negative thoughts are more easily pushed away. They are interfering with your recall pleasure and your sleep so are not welcome at your pillow. After a short time of consistent practice your brain will "get the message".

## THE IMPORTANCE OF A HOBBY
It may be that you face the difficulty of having no hobby; for some reason your life has, perhaps unnoticed, become focused on your job, your business or the very demanding matter of running a house and bringing up the family. Really, this is not very good for you; we all need to have some regular pleasure that we can fall back on, turn to for relief from the undoubted pressures many of us face in day–to–day life. All by itself the lack of a hobby and the relentless tension you may be putting on yourself could explain your sleeplessness.

I believe a hobby is so important that, in case you've fallen out of the habit, in Section Five I have assembled a sample list of hobbies to refresh your memory. When you read it through you will be intrigued to remind yourself of the rich diversity of pastimes you have at your disposal – and there are, no doubt, many others I haven't mentioned.

## BECOME AN EXPERT
Whilst you will not wish to become unhealthily obsessed with your hobby it is certainly worthwhile having in mind the possibility of becoming something of an expert. This will depend upon your youth if you are aiming to become

a dab hand at soccer or athletics, for example, but the older person can, by keen observation of the hobby and study of its records, become quite an authority, even if unable to physically participate. However, as you will see from the list, there are so very many hobbies that active participation is possible for either sex in virtually any age-band.

## FINDING & USING YOUR SLEEP-THOUGHT

For most hobbies there are both specialist magazines and governing bodies/associations. From these you can get dated lists of important events, or champions if your hobby involves competition. By memorising the dated list appropriate to your hobby you construct your positive, pleasing sleep-thought. By silently reciting this list to yourself as you lie comfortably in bed ready to go to sleep you are putting your sleep-thought into action. Every time an unwanted thought tries to intrude concentrate that little bit harder on your sleep-thought. The unwanted thought will go away. You will soon be asleep.

Further on in this chapter I sketch out some hobby sleep-thought examples. First, though, I thought it may be helpful for you to check how I use my own hobby list in my sleep-thought. I have split the list into two parts: the first one I started with was a straight-forward list of the early years of the Men's Singles Championships; date, winner, vanquished and score. I personally never become bored with reciting these bare facts but if you are concerned that such lists would bore *you* (and thus allow negative thoughts to intrude more easily) then you will see a second list in which I set out comments I sometimes recall about each match. Once you have thoroughly mastered your own list you may care to "build in" added tit-bits of interest such as these examples; meantime, stick to basics.

## MY HOBBY LIST AS SLEEP-THOUGHT

This particular list concerns itself with those who have won the Men's Singles at the Lawn Tennis Championships at Wimbledon. I quote just a few of the early years to demonstrate how I immerse myself in my sleep-thought, my hobby, to please myself to sleep.

(For interest, my preferred sleep-preparation position is to lie on my side. Getting the bed-clothes and pillow to my complete satisfaction I then relax my body, paying particular attention to mouth, jaw and throat muscles.) I always begin my sleep-thought by reciting to myself the first year of the Championships, the name of the winner, who he beat and the score:

1877, Spencer William Gore beat William Marshall, 6-1, 6-2, 6-4.
1878, Frank Hadow beat Spencer Gore, 7-5, 6-1, 9-7.
1879, The Reverend John Hartley beat Vere St Leger Goold, 6-2, 6-4, 6-2.
1880, The Reverend John Hartley beat Herbert Lawford, 6-3, 6-2, 2-6, 6-3.
1881, William Renshaw beat The Reverend John Hartley, 6-0, 6-1, 6-1.
1882, William Renshaw beat Ernest Renshaw, 6-1, 2-6, 4-6, 6-2, 6-2.
1883, William Renshaw beat Ernest Renshaw, 2-6, 6-3, 6-3, 4-6, 6-3.

1884, William Renshaw beat Herbert Lawford, 6-0, 6-4, 9-7.
1885, William Renshaw beat Herbert Lawford, 7-5, 6-2, 4-6, 7-5.
1886, William Renshaw beat Herbert Lawford, 6-0, 5-7, 6-3, 6-4.
1887, Herbert Lawford won, William Renshaw defaulting because of injury.

And so on.

## SAMPLE LIST OF COMMENTS FOR OCCASIONAL USE & INTEREST
I will sometimes remind myself of any interesting points about the players or the match itself. Thus something like this:

1877 "Gore was a good rackets player. Funny thing was, this man of tennis history thought lawn tennis was boring."

1878 "Hadow was an even funnier bird than Gore. He was a tea planter on leave and only played to pass the time. He didn't much care for lawn tennis either, went back to his tea planting in Ceylon and didn't bother to return to Wimbledon for 48 years; only then when he was persuaded to come to belatedly receive his Champion's medal. Another rackets player."

1879 "Despite lawn tennis having a vicarage garden image, Hartley was the only vicar ever to win Wimbledon; the irony was that be beat Goold who, some years later, was convicted of murder. Good triumphing over evil."

1880 "This match proved that the vicar was no rabbit; Lawford, who appeared in six finals, ultimately became champion himself in 1887."

1881 "The founding father of the game had arrived. When William Renshaw first won Wimbledon lawn tennis was a pastime. He went on to win the title seven times in all and his skill and fame turned lawn tennis into an international sport."

A few other hobby sleep-thought examples:

## ANOTHER SPORTING THEME
This dated list with a sporting theme concerns venues and nations competing in successive Commonwealth Games. Many sports are involved and you may think of following up on some of them.

| Year | Venue | Sports | Countries Participating |
|---|---|---|---|
| 1930 | Hamilton, Canada | 6 | 11 |
| 1934 | London, England | 6 | 16 |
| 1938 | Sydney, Australia | 7 | 15 |
| 1950 | Auckland, New Zealand | 9 | 12 |
| 1954 | Vancouver, Canada | 9 | 24 |
| 1958 | Cardiff, Wales | 9 | 35 |

| 1962 | Perth, Australia | 9 | 35 |
| 1966 | Kingston, Jamaica | 9 | 34 |
| 1970 | Edinburgh, Scotland | 9 | 42 |
| 1974 | Christchurch, New Zealand | 9 | 39 |
| 1978 | Edmonton, Canada | 10 | 46 |
| 1982 | Brisbane, Australia | 10 | 46 |
| 1986 | Edinburgh, Scotland | 10 | 26 |

## CHINESE ASTROLOGY

On another tack, perhaps Chinese Astrology could interest you (if so, see book noted in Section Five). Whilst our Western horoscopes are based on the solar calendar, Chinese horoscopes are lunar based. It is believed that Buddha named a year after each of those 12 animals who came to bid him farewell before he departed Earth.

We start at 1900 (the year of the "tireless" Rat):

| RAT | 1900 | 1912 | 1924 |
| OX | 1901 | 1913 | 1925 |
| TIGER | 1902 | 1914 | 1926 |
| RABBIT | 1903 | 1915 | 1927 |
| DRAGON | 1904 | 1916 | 1928 |
| SNAKE | 1905 | 1917 | 1929 |
| HORSE | 1906 | 1918 | 1930 |
| SHEEP | 1907 | 1919 | 1931 |
| MONKEY | 1908 | 1920 | 1932 |
| ROOSTER | 1909 | 1921 | 1933 |
| DOG | 1910 | 1922 | 1934 |
| BOAR | 1911 | 1923 | 1935 |

As you see, every 12th year belongs to and is named after the same animal. You may find it an interesting sleep-thought to work out each animal's year by mentally "completing" the columns after 1935, eg, which "year" are we in now? Remember, this is not speculation but fact!

## MALT WHISKY

If your hobby is or could be the appreciation of Single Malt Whisky then here is a sample list in date order of names of just a few of these seductive brews. (Interestingly, the oldest distillery in the world is not Scots, but Irish.) For a more comprehensive list read "Malt Whisky Almanac", details Section Five.

| Date Established | Name | Area Where Made |
|---|---|---|
| 1608 | Bushmills | Country Antrim |
| 1770 | Bowmore | Argyll |
| 1772 | Littlemill | Dumbartonshire |
| 1775 | The Glenlivet | Perthshire |

| 1786 | Strathisla | Banffshire |
| 1794 | Ardberg | Argyll |
| 1795 | Highland Park | Orkney |
| 1798 | Ledaig | Argyll |
| 1800 | Auchentoshan | Dumbartonshire |
| 1804 | Glen Grant | Morayshire |
| 1807 | Milburn | Inverness-shire |
| 1810 | Isle of Jura | Argyll |

## NO LIMITS

There is no limit to the way in which you can use hobbies as sleep-thoughts.
I am sure that either from the above or from the extensive list in Section Five
you will find inspiration. The splendid diversity of human nature guarantees that
some of my readers (perhaps you among them?) will come up with their own
successful variations on my core theme. I would certainly welcome hearing
about them for inclusion in future editions of this booklet.

## A COMPETITION FOR READERS

In the extensive hobby list in Section Five I have put in a very few "hobbies"
that aren't hobbies at all and therefore don't fit into the list. The *first 20 readers*
who write in with the correct list of these non-hobbies, together with some
brief, cogent comments on this booklet, will receive a cheque refunding the
cost of this booklet and a copy of the recent best-seller, "Guide to Village
Riches". (Publishers' decision final.)

## CHAPTER 3:   SOME OPTIONAL AIDS TO GOOD SLEEP

Air Purifier, Baths, Beds, Bed Clothes, Bedroom, Body Heat, Body Relaxation,
Cuddles, Curtains/Eye masks/Fabrics, Earplugs/Double Glazing, Exercise,
Food and Drink, Good Habits, Gurus, Herbs, Music, Nose Drops, Pillows,
Prayer.

Knowing that in some mysterious way sleep will refresh us, we should make
going to bed a pleasure. Unfortunately, failure to get to sleep can, over time,
breed something like dread of bedtime. My sleep formula will cure that but
here are some other ideas that may interest you and make sleep anticipation
more positive and pleasurable.

## AIR PURIFIER

An old recipe is to put a few drops of oil of lavender into a glass of very hot
water, place this on a bedside table and benefit from the permeating fragrance.

## BATHS

As an aid to sleep many swear by a hot bath before retiring but how about a cold one? The Cold Sitz therapy calls for cold water in the bath sufficient to cover your hips and bottom. Wrapping something warm around your upper body, leave the lower half immersed for about 30 seconds before drying off. The Sitz is said to bring peace and relaxation by drawing the body energy away from the head. Whatever temperature of bath you choose be ready to retire immediately after bathing.

## BEDS

Have a good look at your existing bed with a view to upgrading it. A cheap and/or ancient bed may not be helping you get proper sleep, particularly if it is also the wrong size for you. The ideal size of bed should be six inches longer than you are tall and at least three foot six inches wide. Big is better for your bed; only then will you relax (instead of perhaps worrying about falling off it in your sleep!).

## BED CLOTHES

I recommend a duvet, preferably filled and covered with natural materials; big enough to really enfold you in a soothing, snug embrace. Consider, in addition, a pure fleece under-blanket.

## THE BEDROOM ITSELF

As you suffer from poor sleep you may be particularly sensitive to the atmosphere around you. I believe that buildings and their rooms do give off an aura (the Chinese call it Ch'i, or cosmic breath). If this proposition makes sense to you then have a careful look at your bedroom layout to ensure that the furniture, and most particularly your bed, is in the most "comfortable" Ch'i position in the room.

Ideally, the bed should be in a "protected" part of the bedroom, eg, I have found that beds opposite doors or under windows can bring a lack of ease.

I suggest that it is not a good idea to use your bedroom for reading, eating, watching TV, etc. Try hard to make your bedroom a temple to sleep so that this goal dominates your thoughts when you enter.

## BODY HEAT

We vary in our response to bedroom temperatures. It's worth erring on the side of having the bedroom cooler (but not draughty; have you insulated your loft?) rather than hotter, but, as we lose heat from our head (hands and feet, too, if they escape from under the bed covers), don't be above the idea of using a nightcap, mittens and bedsocks if these will keep you more comfortable in colder weather.

## BODY RELAXATION

Physical relaxation promotes mental calm. The following routine is therefore a useful prelude to normal sleep when you settle down at night. The object is complete relaxation of voluntary muscles to enable reduction of waste products produced by their activity, and to reduce oxygen demands.

Lay your hands across your abdomen, with the fingers lightly interlaced, arms resting on the bed. Breathe in deeply, filling the abdomen first (diaphragmatic breathing) and then sigh out and repeat this a few times, audibly if it helps.

Now, allow the breathing to continue at its own pace and depth, but, as you sigh out, concentrate on one part of your body, letting go with each breath. Start with the ankles and feet, letting them flop outwards where gravity takes them. Feel the joints loosening. Move on to the legs for the next breath or two and work up your body, conveying the idea of letting go as you come to each part, even if at first it won't quite relax as well as you would like it to.

Once you feel that ankles, calves and knees are relaxed forget them and move up in this order:
- hips and thighs: think particularly of the inner thigh muscles which are often tense as subconscious protectors of the genital organs;
- hands and forearms: feel the small muscles and joints in the fingers relaxing;
- abdomen: let it sag;
- chest: feel the muscles between the ribs letting go;
- the whole back, from the buttocks up to the shoulders: feel them sinking and spreading on the bed;
- neck and shoulders: often difficult to let go but send the message through and it will eventually get there;
- head and face: feel the eyes sinking back into their sockets, jaw muscles slacken, mouth relax.
- don't forget the tiniest muscle of all; if you can mentally "reach" it, you may actually feel the stapedius muscle in the middle ear relax.

With one or two deeper breaths and sighs feel the whole body sinking into deeper relaxation – sigh . . . sink . . . and sag.

Let your breathing proceed at it's own pace; it will sometimes slow right down, or occasionally a deeper sigh will want to come through. Allow any muscular twitches and jerks to take their course. They are just due to tension being released.

Now proceed to your pleasurable sleep-thought and very soon you will be asleep.

**CUDDLES**
Whether you get yours from a loved one, your dog or even a soft cuddly toy there is widespread agreement that cuddles are a most enjoyable aid to sleep. No, it's not soppy; it's sane! (See the book noted in Section Five Information Check List.)

## CURTAINS/EYE MASKS/FABRICS

I find eye masks uncomfortable, only to be used when there is nothing to be done about intrusive light. In your own bedroom, of course, you can curtain windows, even doors, against light. I take this concern with total bedroom darkness even further by actually travelling with window curtains in case I find myself in a room where light filters in. (Far too many hotels fail to give any thought to this menace.) Close-weave black cotton is the saviour material and several thicknesses may be necessary. For travel, the material neatly folds up to a handleable size for packing. Available from curtain shops are other, opaque, lighter-coloured fabrics to coordinate with bedroom decor.

For bed clothes, night gowns and other fabrics intimate to you I recommend natural cotton or wool. Synthetics can set up allergies.

## EARPLUGS/DOUBLE GLAZING

For years I have used Boots' "Muffles", the cheapest, most effective and comfortable earplugs and although I can sleep without them I am much more content with. However, I am in a quiet environment; if you have the misfortune to sleep in a noisy one but don't care for earplugs then the cost of bedroom double-glazing may not be too high a price to pay for peace and quiet. Whilst a boon, wax earplugs are a bit fiddly — you must spend a few minutes kneading them soft, then shaping them to your ear (cut them down to size if necessary if you have small ears). DO NOT make them too small or you could have difficulty removing them.

## EXERCISE

As yet sleep scientists have not shown a very clear relationship between exercise and quality sleep; the decision therefore must be an individual one: if you are not exercising at all should you try a modest amount? If you are already taking exercise should you increase this?

There is undoubtedly wide agreement that exercise is a "good thing". I would base my cautious support for it on the proposal that if sensible exercise can help to get others healthily tired and more ready for sleep then perhaps you should experiment to see if this is true *for you*.

If you decide to exercise don't overdo it. Better still, join a peer group and get professional advice from a qualified instructor. If exercise turns out to be good for you it will also help to take you out of yourself and get any problems into perspective.

I recommend you do not over-stimulate your body with exercise just before bed.

(My own exercise? Two miles walking each day with the dogs. Heaven!)

## FOOD AND DRINK

As I have said in Chapter One, it is important to leave at least two hours between any evening meal and sleep-time. If you have consistent difficulty in leaving enough time to digest the food then consider either a change in routine (are you working too late?) or even switching your main meal to lunch time. You may have to avoid some "heavy" foods (red meat, spiced meals, curries, fried food, even such things as bananas, nuts and cheese) which take between four and six hours to digest. Unless you can finish them well before you go to bed, you'll be better off with fish, poultry and lightly steamed vegetables.

If for any reason bedtime arrives and you haven't eaten then content yourself with some Horlicks or Ovaltine and biscuits and make up the food shortfall the next day if you feel really hungry.

How healthy we are is largely determined by what we put into our bodies and, if you're interested in a long life as well as a well-slept one, you'll want to know that students of mankind have noted that societies renowned for longevity all have one thing in common – their citizens ate very little.

As we drink tea and coffee for the "lift" they give us they are not ideal bedtime drinks. Herbal drinks are okay but alternatively consider milk as a night-cap. It soothes because it contains an amino acid (Tryptophan) which forms the body's natural sedative (Serotonin). Incidentally, if tea's your favourite brew you might try making it with milk, not water. An old recipe claims that this removes the tannic acid; however, the stimulant caffeine will still be there, even if "damped down".

My view on diet is this: Only take corrective action if something seems wrong or goes wrong. It may be that a little less of this, more of that, will bring you back to rights. Only if this self-healing fails should expert advice be sought.

Taking responsibility for our own health is very much the mood of the 90's and the success of this movement to a large extent will depend on common sense and, indeed, scepticism, particularly about every food fad and scare. Regrettably, these have become almost daily features of modern life.

## GOOD HABITS

Many pundits have written in praise of "the automatic reaction to a specific situation", or habit. The American politician T. B. Reed suggested that "For the ordinary business of life, an ounce of habit is worth a pound of intellect".

As this book is based on the good habit idea, I naturally believe that there is a powerful case in favour of building a whole set of positive habits upon which to run our lives. After all, why not consign many of our recurrent and essential functions to the automode of habit? Are you improved in any way by, for example, having to daily make a conscious decision as to when to have a bowel movement? Consider what happens when this critical function is left random: The body suffers because it is getting clogged with waste it must get rid of; the mind works less well because of the body's below-par functioning.

Consider replacing this randomness with a simply-learned habit: Train yourself to go straight to the lavatory as soon as you've had your morning cuppa (preferably hot). For the first few days perhaps nothing will happen; stick to the habit for a week and you will find your bowels responding – automatically. Result: you begin your day refreshed, your body fit, your mind freed to get on with other important, creative matters.

As good daily habits accumulate you are all the time further assuring yourself of a good night's sleep, for, as you have seen, that too can be achieved by habit. Also, what do they say about winning? Why, of course – it's a habit!

## GURUS and ALTERNATIVE THERAPIES
In a therapy booklet which unavoidably has to address problems it may be useful to refer to the many problem-solvers on offer. Whilst I am quite sure that this book will get you back to quality sleep, it may be that you will feel the need for some outside assistance in particular areas; if so you will find a short sample list of sources in Section Five.

## HERBS
Essential for bringing unique flavour to our cooking, herbs have since ancient times been rightly prized for their medicinal properties. Try to avoid tablets – go for the natural, fresh product wherever possible to benefit fully from its gentle, soothing healing. See Section Five for a book that will show you how to get the best from the plants, e.g. although there are times when only the "hard" drinks (tea, coffee) will do to give that needed kick-start, I am experimenting with herb teas and find that they do appear to help towards clarity and calm.

Some people are devoted to another herby idea, herb-filled pillows. See Section Five for makers, who claim that natural body warmth releases the aromatic essences so that you breathe them in whilst sleeping. One pillow is meant to encourage sleep, the other to unblock your nose! Before you buy it may be a good idea to test that you're not allergic to any of the herbs.

## MUSIC
There is support for the idea of using music to help get you to sleep. If you have a favourite composer then why not invite him or her into your bedroom? I suggest that earphones (which will disturb comfortable movement of your head on the pillow) and violent music would be counter-productive but, as most of the higher forms of music rely upon soothing rhythms and harmonies, these sounds may be helpful in pleasing you, thus getting you relaxed for

quality sleep. (However, guard against the music stopping whilst you're still awake!)

## NOSE DROPS

As an occasional sleep aid nose drops are useful because a blocked nose may awaken you during the night and hinder your return to sleep. If you have this problem, get your doctor to examine you and it may be that he will prescribe a decongestant. If he does not feel that the problem justifies a prescription but you are still troubled then an over-the-counter decongestant that is effective is Otrivine. However, long term use of nose drops is not recommended, so if you're using them most nights you will have to find a cure for the underlying problem. (Also see Chapter Six on SNORING).

## PILLOWS

Another important item where the sheer sense of well-being will make a good pillow (with natural filling if possible) a worthwhile investment. You may be baffled by orthopaedic pillows; there are many on the market and just any old one may not be the one for you, eg, you will require a different thickness of pillow according to your size. Noted in Section Five the ones that my wife and I use. Also see HERBS for other pillow ideas.

## PRAYER

Not for everyone, but I believe that it puts you into calmer frame of mind immediately prior to sleep. As prayer enables us to thank loved ones (and perhaps helps ease those little twinges of guilt?), re-affirm our beliefs and focus minds on a better future, it has all the positive features so essential to sleep-preparation.

# SECTION TWO

**Chapter 4:  Sleeping, Dreaming & Science:
Do The Mysteries Linger On?**

---

## CHAPTER 4:  SLEEPING, DREAMING & SCIENCE: DO THE MYSTERIES LINGER ON?

Now that you know how your sleeplessness is going to be cured you will probably be interested in this brief sketch of sleep from the scientific viewpoint.

The short answer to the question in this chapter heading is – "yes".

However, whilst our knowledge is far from complete, we do know more now than we did; the breakthrough came in the 1960's with the beginning of the use of the EEG (electro-encephalograph, a device for detecting and recording the electrical activity of the brain). Sleep laboratories sprang up and soon began to find out more about the mysteries of sleep and dreaming that have fascinated us since ancient times. Here are just some of the many points of interest that have emerged:

### A GENERAL SLEEP PATTERN

Most of us conform to a general sleep pattern which reads something like this: Following drowsiness, we drift into what is called Stage One Sleep. This light sleep lasts only a short time (up to 10 minutes) before normally being overtaken by Stages Two, Three and Four, which each in turn denotes a progressively deeper state of sleep.

These first four stages are known as slow wave (or orthodox) sleep stages to distinguish them from REM (Rapid Eye Movement) sleep which is identified by its very different brainwave, the observable movement of the eyes under the closed lids and the loss of neck muscle tone; this syndrome is referred to as "paradoxical" sleep. REM sleep will arrive approximately 45 minutes after sleep starts. Its first session will typically occupy almost 15 minutes before the sleeper returns to orthodox sleep and the process will be repeated, with variations, throughout the night's sleep. As the night progresses individual REM sleep sessions may extend for up to a half-hour.

### DREAMING & AVERAGE SLEEP TIMES

Whilst dreaming may happen in orthodox sleep stages, it seems that REM sleep sessions are the ones that are dominated by dreams and, awoken in the middle of REM sleep, the dreamer may be able to report the most recent part of the dream but otherwise dreams are quickly forgotten. Scientists believe that dreams actually occupy as much real time as it takes you to dream them; apparently they are not "concertina'd", as had been theorised previously.

Although, of course, actual sleep times vary, the average time slept by a healthy young adult comes out at about 7½ hours per night, of which time approximately half is spent in light sleep, one quarter in deep sleep and one quarter in REM sleep. When very young we sleep much more, when elderly somewhat less than average.

## SHORT SLEEP, NON-SLEEP & TOO MUCH SLEEP

There is a significant minority who are very happy and healthy with much less sleep than usual. Former Prime Minister, Mrs Thatcher, is reputed to sleep between only three and five hours per night and trained herself to these spartan hours in order to cope with her awesome schedule. The Mrs Thatchers of this world do not waste time on light sleep stages, however. With typical forthrightness they get rapidly to deep sleep Stage Four and REM sleep, which together occupy almost their entire sleeping time. (This has caused some scientists to wonder about the function of light sleep.)

On record is another lady who gets along very contentedly on an average of one hour's sleep per night. However, nobody has been discovered who survives indefinitely without any sleep. Scientists are sceptical of reported cases of people who claim not to sleep at all and those that have been laboratory-tested nodded off at some point. The longest recorded period of voluntary "sleeplessness" took place in 1986; the subject is alleged to have remained awake for over 453 hours, or nearly 19 complete days.

In extended periods of enforced sleeplessness, the "drive" towards sleep becomes dominant; so powerful that other "drives" (to food, sex, etc) are increasingly submerged. Whilst apparently active during lengthy periods awake, test subjects have been observed to take micro-naps to keep them going.

Whilst many people believe they need nine or even more hours sleep per night, too much sleep seems to create similar problems to those experienced by people getting too little, eg, calculation, vigilance and co-ordination all suffer noticeably. However, deprived of sleep, hallucinations and mounting incoherence feature.

## SLEEP "LEARNING", "INSPIRATION" & TIME MONITORING

The chances are poor of successfully learning something (for example, a language or skill) whilst asleep. However, there are reports of some remarkable "inspirations" following sleep, although it is noted that such revelations are usually preceded by intense conscious thought, with sleep perhaps being the "key" that unlocks and opens the door to seeing a solution. (I myself have noticed that if I give a problem some careful thought then consign it to my "compost heap" of the subconscious then, overnight, or within a few days, a solution will often surface. But what role does sleep actually play in all of this? I wish I knew. Sometimes the "method" seems to work, though.)

It seems certain that people can "programme" themselves to wake at fairly precise times; apparently we can, and do, monitor time in some way whilst asleep.

## INSOMNIACS
Apparently, insomniacs are not always to be relied upon to give accurate reports on their sleeplessness. It is not uncommon for subjects to report broken sleep despite EEG recordings and visual observations that show sleep to have been normal.

Research indicates that insomniacs may have certain things in common: they may be sleeping at the wrong time and seeking to sleep longer than they really need; they may have unrealistic expectations of their sleep; they are likely to have an underlying anxiety that is behind the sleeplessness and they are likely to dwell excessively upon their problem, with resentment and anger arising, which disrupt sleep.

Devising and sticking to a pre-sleep routine whilst experimenting to discover actual, not supposed, sleep needs; forgiving enemies and counting blessings are amongst the insomnia remedies suggested.

Despite the rather gloomy news that 50% of the UK population complain about insomnia at one time or another, sleep scientists appear to feel that there are very few totally intractable sleep problems.

## SLEEP AND CONVENTION
Animals and very young and very old humans take their sleep in several chunks throughout the 24 hours. Those of us who take sleep all at once, scientists think, are conforming to a culture geared to day-time activity (such as jobs, getting children to and from school, etc) and night-time rest. Whether it is entirely "natural" or beneficial for us to take our sleep in this way remains a matter of conjecture. A test, in which a subject mimicked Leonardo da Vinci's sleep patterns, found no impairment of mental and physical performance. For three weeks the 27-year-old subject slept for just two-and-a-half hours per day in six, 25-minute spells.

Another theory is that the human is "programmed" to have *two* bouts of sleep per 24-hour cycle!

## SLEEP AS A HEALTH BAROMETER
American studies have indicated a link exists between how long we sleep each night and how long we live. Researchers believe that older people who sleep more than 10½ hours or less than 4½ hours per night may be experiencing "pathological sleep", indicating that their health is in danger. Support stems

from the fact that disease, such as cancer or cardiac disorder, is preceded by abnormally long or short sleep patterns. Further study may enable sleep disorders to be related to the development of specific diseases, thus foreseeing and perhaps delaying death.

## SUBSTANCES THAT MAY CAUSE SLEEP AND WAKING
Scientists hope they have discovered the body substances that trigger the slide from consciousness to sleep, and that regulate waking up. One substance, called Prostaglandin $D_2$, scientists say, induces sleep; the other, Prostaglandin $E_2$, was found to induce and maintain wakefulness. If proven, these discoveries will have profound effects on and give new insights into sleep and its disorders. Nevertheless, because Prostaglandins have multiple roles in bodily functions, the manufacture of, for example, sleeping and waking pills made from these substances will have to be very finely focused before they can become an effective reality. This "will take a very long time."

## BUT WHAT ARE SLEEP AND DREAMS FOR?
Sleep researchers have learned and are learning much but they still admit that they do not know what sleep and dreaming are actually *for*. But they have some theories: Because of the hectic activity observed during Rapid Eye Movement sleep, which brings it closer to wakefulness than sleep, some scientific opinion is tending towards a belief that slow wave (stages 1-4) sleep and REM sleep are serving quite different functions. They speculate that slow wave sleep represents the time when the body refreshes and repairs itself, and that REM sleep sessions are used to repair the brain and maintain the central nervous system, eg, excessive alcohol intake is believed to "block" REM sleep; this may explain next day "hangovers," during which we find our mental functions to be below par, presumably because the brain has been unable to adequately repair itself overnight.

As to the predominantly REM-activated dreams, there is considerable scientific scepticism that they have any useful meaning; dream "interpretation" (including Freud's weighty views supporting it) is largely discredited. Rather does some opinion favour the idea that dreams are simply the brain's method of "clearing the decks", getting rid of valueless mental junk! Nevertheless, some psychotherapy still concerns itself with dreams, not so much with the intention of "interpreting" them but rather to gain some insight into what is going on in the patient's mind and what may be pre-occupying him.

Interestingly, scientists think that during a dream we are *completely* single-minded and that the imagery of the dream dominates and excludes imagination and intention. The theory goes that as we cannot "make notes" and form the intention to remember dreams are consequently ephemeral. This appears to support the perception that the brain has the ability to "shut out" anything that it does not wish to entertain. However, it does not explain how we are able to recall all or some of our dreams.

Whatever the use of dreams, tests on animals indicate that they, too, appear to dream. (Watch and listen to your dog or cat when they're going through a REM sleep session!).

Some idea of the magnitude of the task facing sleep researchers can be found when contemplating the enigma of two-headed human monsters. It has been noted that one "twin" may seem fast asleep whilst the "other" is wide awake. This despite their sharing the same body system.!

## QUALITY SLEEP: THE NEW THERAPY

Americans are increasingly turning away from psychotherapy and towards sleep therapy to resolve their problems as conviction finally and, in my view, belatedly, takes root that quality sleep is absolutely essential to a good life. This movement is strengthened because it is believed that lack of sleep was the cause of some major problems such as the Challenger space shuttle disaster, the Three Mile Island nuclear power accident and the Chernobyl catastrophe. As a result of these perceptions almost every major American hospital has a sleep clinic for patients; despite the evidence that there are millions of sufferers here, the UK has only 14 hospitals with such clinics and a mere handful of specially equipped sleep laboratories.

## SLEEP SCIENCE AND THE FUTURE

Sleep research has moved out of the foothills but has still a hard slog ahead of it – eg, there are apparently some 80 medical sleep disorder categories – so surely common sense will convince us that we ought to be doing more to help fund the sleep scientists in their search for the answers?

Meantime, the mysteries do linger on: what are sleeping and dreaming really *for*?

Whilst the search for answers continues, take this advice: get your share of sleep. In an average lifetime we can spend up to 25 years in bed slumbering; if sometime in the future the boffins were to prove that we actually don't need to sleep at all, it may occur to somebody in power to make us put all that "redundant" sleep time to productive use!

# SECTION THREE

---

## CHAPTER 5:    PILLS: DRUGGED BODIES ARE PARALYSED, NOT RESTED

Although your GP may give compelling reasons for putting you on tranquillisers and/or sleeping pills there are two general guides to bear in mind: (a) such drugs should only usually be taken in the very short term, and (b) an holistic practitioner is unlikely ever to recommend them. Here's why:-

**THESE PILLS ARE NOT USER-FRIENDLY**
These drugs have at least two negative properties in common: They are addictive and therefore capable of abuse and, as no drug has ever been devised that has only one action, they carry side-effects, some of them extremely unpleasant.

For many doctors, prescribing sleeping pills and tranquillisers is often an available "solution" to an otherwise "intractable" problem, but the exercise in the medium and long-term can be self-defeating. I quote much of the following from "The Tranquilliser Trap", a booklet from a charity called Natural Medicines Society (for further details see Section Five):
1.   Benzodiazepanes are widely used as sleeping pills and tranquillisers and it is estimated that, in the UK alone, three million people have become addicted to them.
2.   Despite the above, millions of prescriptions are still handed out every year.
3.   The long list of side-effects found to occur during use is frightening. Here are just a few: fearfulness, suicidal tendencies, confusion, depression, anxiety, personality change, giddiness, anger and *insomnia*. Long-term use of tranquillisers can cause brain damage.
4.   Ironically, sleeping pills actually start to *cause* sleeplessness after a very short period. NMS estimate they cease to be beneficial between three and 14 days after use commences. Side-effects begin to show during even this short time.

5.  When addiction occurs withdrawal is a difficult business, eg, NMS report that "coming off" Ativan is said to be worse than withdrawing from heroin; in extreme cases doctors have to prescribe Valium to help sufferers withdraw from Ativan. NMS counsel that withdrawal should only be gradual and, ideally, done with qualified help. They warn of the many withdrawal symptoms, just a few of which include: panic attacks, feelings of unreality, loss of memory, loss of libido, nausea, urinary problems and *insomnia* (see below).

## HELP FROM YOUR ADVISER

What is to be done? For those afflicted by these drugs the road ahead is clearly difficult, but the problem is too pernicious to be left in limbo. A start must be made with your doctor; he can be your most valuable ally if sympathetic to your request to begin withdrawal. If unsympathetic, then a second medical opinion should be sought. There may be serious reasons why your continued use of the drugs is absolutely essential; if not, and your doctor(s) will not help, then you should seek help from an holistic practitioner.

## TAKE STOCK, THEN ACTION

Where drugs are being taken continually to alleviate some unhappiness it is worth reflecting that the unhappiness may well be there to force you to take stock, to get to the root of the sadness. This cannot happen if the difficulty is continuously being masked, and probably distorted, by the drugs.

Clearly, common sense dictates that *drug-free,* quality sleep must be the aim. As noted in 3 above, if you have been taking these drugs you may have had insomnia, regardless. By taking a withdrawal course and practising my sleep formula you will quite quickly eliminate any insomnia whilst assuring yourself that you are at last on the safe and *natural* road back to a normal and contented life.

# CHAPTER 6:   SNORING: SOME CAUSES & CURES

It has been estimated that one person in eight snores regularly. Some snores have been recorded at 90 decibels, equivalent to the din put out by a fire alarm. Experts say that snoring can and does wreck marriages, cause law suits and bankrupt businesses. Is snoring an audible cry for help? Perhaps, and if so all is not lost. There are cures but before detailing these it might be helpful to examine what we know about the condition.

## SOME REASONS FOR SNORING

We recognise a snore as a hoarse "rattling" or grunting noise and one of the causes is that the muscles of our soft palate and throat relax in sleep and, as we breathe, the thin edges of the palate vibrate like the reed in a wood-wind instrument.

Whilst you can snore when the mouth is closed there is no doubt, nevertheless, that nature intends that we should breathe through the nose because (a) the smell-perceiving cells are high up in the nasal cavity so air breathed in through the nose can be monitored for quality; (b) the nose has a built-in air filter in the form of those coarse nostril hairs which trap dust that otherwise might irritate the delicate lining of the lungs; (c) the blood which supplies the mucus membrane inside the nose warms incoming air to a temperature comfortable to the body.

Of course, if the nasal passages become blocked then snoring is again likely to result. The blockages can be transitory – mucus from smoking (see below), a cold or hayfever, etc; or structural, where, for example, the partition between the nostrils (the septum) has become distorted, perhaps due to an external blow.

If the difficulty of breathing through the nose becomes too great then nature's response, of course, is to compel us to breathe through the mouth, at which point the uvula (that little piece of flesh that hangs free at the rear of the soft palate helping to stop food going up into the nose), together with the soft palate's edges, reverberate noisily like reed instruments in the draught. Result: snoring.

The ideal physical position for a good snore is sleeping on the back. Even with none of the other conditions mentioned above, sleeping in this way can cause the tongue to flop back, impeding the airway. Snoring may again result.

## THOSE WHO MAY SNORE
Who is likely to be a snorer?

## DRINKERS
Alcohol gets to the brain very fast and, in excess, will effect the command mechanisms controlling muscle relaxation and breathing regularity. If the drinker also smokes then the problem is compounded.

## THE OBESE
Obesity is the term generally applied where a person weighs 20% or more in excess of the ideal weight. This condition makes the victim more vulnerable to a wide variety of ailments, including a proneness to physical accidents. This last perhaps provides a clue to their snoring: faulty co-ordination can lead to breathing difficulties. Another theory is that excessive fat causes the throat to become narrower, making breathing more laboured and noisy.

Perhaps the most likely explanation is that, because of their bulk, fat people will tend more than normally-shaped people to wind up sleeping on their back, the perfect pre-condition for most snoring.

## SMOKERS
The smoker is quite likely to be a snorer. Cigarette smoke is an irritant and thus causes inflammation; the body responds to this threat by increasing mucus production. (Because of "passive smoking" a smoker's non-smoking partner could also be a snorer!)

## THE UNWELL
Illnesses likely to cause snoring range from the common cold, hayfever, asthma, infected tonsils and adenoids to bronchitis, pneumonia, TB and lung cancer.

A very special case of being unwell is known as Sleep Apnea in which breathing is paralysed during sleep by loose flaps of tissue blocking the airway. The build-up of carbon monoxide in the blood that this causes leads to periodic explosive grunting and gasping for air. Although the sufferer will awaken each time this happens, the waking periods, although numerous, can be so brief that the victim may not be aware of them but, because of the disruption to sleep, will certainly feel sleepy during the day. In addition, apnea victims are likely to have problems with long-distance car-driving; falling asleep at the wheel due to chronic tiredness is not unknown.

For what is known as Central Sleep Apnea (where an innate central nervous system malfunction may be the cause) no cure is available.

## TEMPORARY SNORERS
May include those who, for example, have had to undergo surgery after which sleeping on the back is difficult or impossible to avoid during recuperation. After recovery the snoring should cease when normal on-the-side sleeping is resumed.

## SNORING CURES
Pretty clearly snoring causes wide-spread distress and chaos and must be taken very seriously; every cure, however way out, should be considered with care. What's on offer? Although snorers cannot escape the consequences of their unfortunate and involuntary uproar, I've tried to "grade" the cures from minimally inconvenient to more drastic remedies.
1.    Experiment with some nose drops, eg, Otrivine (over the chemist's counter) or Dexarhinaspray (prescription). However, if nose drops do work you will still have to correct the underlying difficulty because you cannot take nose drops every night without possibly causing other problems. See also Section Five re a book on essential oils that can ease respiratory problems.
2.    An ear, nose and throat consultant has developed "Snorestop", a moulded pillow which has a cavity in the middle and, as the back of the head sinks

into this, the neck is gently extended to aid normal breathing. Users claim that, after a few nights getting used to it, they get a better night's sleep. As importantly, partners report a reduction in snoring.

3. "Snore No More" is a micro-electronic device shaped and worn like a large wrist watch. When it picks up the distinctive sound waves of your snoring it triggers a tiny electric charge to the skin, insufficient to hurt or wake you but enough to make you shift position so that your snoring mode is disturbed and, hopefully, stopped.

4. Less comfortable but certainly cheap is the idea of sewing something onto the back of nightclothes. A cotton reel, possibly a ping pong ball, will deter the snorer from sleeping on his back.

5. Some dieticians suggest that a look at your diet may be rewarding. For instance, dairy products are said to be mucus-inducing if taken to excess, as well as being at the root of various allergies. See the books mentioned in the Information Check List, Chapter One, Section Five.

6. Consider another expert tip: keeping the mouth shut by sticky-taping the lower jaw onto both cheeks. Not a joke; it's said to work.

7. Sleep experts have now devised a snore-prevention, hi-tech mask to be worn to bed. The mask is attached to an air blower and the air pressure keeps open the snorer's airways. Although snorers report good results, with better sleep and an improvement in their waking lives, the experts warn that it is "inconvenient" to wear. If the problem is that serious yet cannot be solved by the other, simpler methods mentioned, the snorer probably has an obligation to try what sounds like a sure-fire cure, in the short term. However, as being permanently on an air blower cannot be acceptable, see my comments in 9 below.

8. Another radical "solution" is to isolate the snorer in a separate bedroom. Sad to say, this social deprivation may be accompanied by financial expense: there's plenty of evidence that really serious snorers need to sleep in professionally sound-proofed rooms!

9. If air blowers and separate bedrooms are unacceptable then the painful path of rooting out the underlying cause of the snoring lies ahead: apart from a careful study of diet as suggested in 5 above, if the snoring is related to smoking, alcohol or obesity, for example, then a fairly drastic change of lifestyle will be involved. (See Section Five). Also you may need professional help, in which case your first visit should be to your GP or holistic advisor who can refer you to specialists if necessary.

10. I referred to Apnea: whilst it is regrettably true that Central Sleep Apnea has no current remedy, that caused by loose tissue flapping over and blocking the airway can be completely cured by surgery. Similarly, if bad tonsils and adenoids are causing snoring then they can be surgically treated which should stop the problem.

## VICTIMS CAN HELP AND BE HELPED

The trouble is, of course, that the person best able to throw light on the snoring is asleep whilst he's doing it, so the effectiveness of a cure is usually going to depend upon a second party staying awake and monitoring the results of snore-cure experiments. That said, snoring can be stopped if the parties concerned are determined to explore every avenue until the appropriate cure is found.

You will recall that in Chapter Three I suggested using wax earplugs as a desirable sleep aid option. However, for the afflicted partner of a snorer, the use of earplugs is, in my opinion, absolutely essential. They can dramatically lessen the noise impact and give significant relief whilst a cure is being found. It is also probable that, although normally a quality sleeper, a snorer's partner will find that he or she has to use my sleep formula to assist in getting back to sleep after being awakened by the din.


# CHAPTER 7:  HOW TO FACE & BEAT THE
#                          SLEEP-WRECKERS

As noted in Chapter One, 50% of us are said to suffer from sleep problems. Whilst my sleep formula will get you to sleep, it makes sense to try and ensure the best quality slumber; this can be achieved by facing, then removing nagging worries wherever possible. Below you will a solution-finding method that will help.

Poor sleep affects your judgement and perspective, two qualities that need to be at their best if you are to successfully solve a personal problem. Therefore, take early steps to master my sleep formula before you begin to seek solutions.

The method is as follows:
- Whilst you are getting your sleep right try to increase concentration on day-time activities. As there is a big difference between worrying and calm deliberation, don't "dwell" on or fret over the problem. BE HERE NOW.
- When you're ready to seek a solution (and please don't delay unduly), try if possible to do it away from the distractions of your day-to-day environment. If you have someone you trust and respect to talk things through with this is a great bonus. (For some people a second party is vital.)
- Try to assess your difficulty in a slightly different light; stop viewing it only as a negative – start to see the search for a solution as a positive *challenge* to your ingenuity.
- If you don't correctly identify your problem then obviously you will fail to solve it, so track the beast right to its lair. Look at the difficulty really hard, then ask yourself what it is you fear about it. Keep asking until you know the answer.
- There are often other solutions than just "black" or "white". Write these other solutions down, however way out they may appear; eg, if emigrating

to Outer Mongolia would solve your dilemma, write it down.

- Weigh your options; obviously you want the best solution but don't insist on only the ideal. Consider compromise.
- Write out your eventual, chosen solution – in detail, including dates for completing each step.
- Put your plan into *early* action and try your utmost to stick tight to it.
- Check on your dates and evaluate the success or otherwise as these dates arrive. If you fail, don't give up – you will probably have learned sufficient to devise a new solution that *will* work.

Some further ideas about problem-solving:

**FLOATING TO A SOLUTION**
Whatever your problem it is likely that some sessions in a Floatation Tank will benefit you. Float Therapy involves bobbing quietly about on the surface of water saturated with Epsom Salts. The 60-minute sessions take place in a darkened tank located at a FT centre. FT users find that the therapy not only soothes body aches but also induces great mental calm. FT therapy is claimed to help numerous addictions and ills, including smoking, other drug addictions and insomnia. Get location details from Section Five.

**ARE DOCTORS THE ONLY HOPE?**
Throughout this booklet, and where you a have a choice, I have made reference to seeing your GP *or* holistic therapist. It is essential to have this choice because some doctors never seem to have, or make, the time to delve into and help solve those various problems that cause great mental stress and unhappiness and leave one feeling below-par; you may get a prescription but often don't get a cure! To find out why this is, and what you might do about it, read "The Health Crisis" (details in Section Five). Stubborn problems will not always be solved by medicines or drugs; holistic therapy looks at the complete person and his lifestyle; treatment is based on this holistic appraisal, not just on surface symptons. Perhaps you may need this kind of assistance as opposed to the narrower, more orthodox treatments generally available. Consider.

**LAUGHTER**
If you can see your problem as a challenge you may have prepared yourself to employ perhaps the most valuable weapon of all – LAUGHTER (see Section Five). Before you dismiss this idea as inappropriate to the seriousness of your difficulty see also my comments on PAIN (Chapter Eight and Section Five). Even facing the most serious challenge of all, laughter has a vital, indeed even life-saving, part to play.

**A CHINESE VIEW OF PROBLEMS**
 A Chinese sage once remarked: "When I think I have a trouble I try to send it away. If it will not go I sigh and then take this troublesome trouble along to that place where all the world's troubles are piled high. I gaze on this

mountain of woe and then I look hard to find my own trouble but often it has taken itself off, ashamed of its emptiness."

If comparing our troubles to other people's is a useful therapy then maybe these statistics will help:

## SUFFERING AND HAPPINESS

- Approximately 70 million Europeans and the same number of Americans suffer from sleep disorders.
- Estimates vary but between 10% and 16% of all UK visits to the doctor are said to be about insomnia.
- American women are more than twice as likely as men to be chronic worriers. In the UK studies show than men and women are more sharing – they worry 50–50.
- A recent UK survey suggested that over 50% of women feel tired all of the time. Of these 90% were under 40 years of age.
- A recent report on "How Stressful Is Your Job?" found that, on a scale 1 to 10, the least stressful was that of a museum worker (2). Policemen/women (7.7) and miners (8.3) headed up the list, perceiving theirs as the most stressful jobs.
- Happiest at work? A survey showed clergymen as the most content, rating their degree of job satisfaction at 58% out of 100.
- Least happy, with only 11%, were actuaries – the people who compile statistics!

## CHAPTER 8:   SLEEP ODDITIES

**CHURCHILL'S KNACK**
So-called because war-time premier Winston Churchill coped with the strain
by training himself to go fast asleep for short periods whenever opportunity
arose; eg, he usually slept on the trip from 10 Downing Street to the House
of Commons. Journey time? Less than five minutes! (Got a new-born baby?
Then you may find Churchill's Knack useful: Unlike everybody else, the new
arrival has no sleep pattern at all for the first 12 months so parents will be up
and down at all hours.)

**DRINKING**
If you think that a good old drinking binge will drown your worries and
make you sleep well then better think again: You will get off to sleep more
quickly than normal but may find that you get what is called a "rebound", ie
once the alcohol is "burned off" (metabolised) by the body you are likely to
waken just a few short hours later and have difficulty getting back to sleep
again.

**HEAD-BANGING**
More young children than you might think prepare themselves for sleep by
rhythmically banging their head on their pillow; some even bang against an
adjacent hard surface such as a wall. Although the practice appears rather
alarming, parents should not deter it (difficult, anyway) unless it is evident
that the banging is becoming hard enough to cause injury. This is unlikely. It
is not a good idea to pad any hard surface used by the child; the impact he
intuitively needs is the one that he's getting! If the noise disturbs then better
to rearrange the bedroom if possible. In most cases the practice is harmless
and will pass with childhood.

**NIGHT TERRORS & NIGHTMARES**
Although mainly associated with childhood, nightmares particularly can
continue into adult life. These conditions may be symptoms of the sufferer
attempting to resolve an underlying conflict and so could need skilled analysis.
Immediately after an attack the sufferer can be calmed and helped back to
sleep by stroking the right forearm with the fingertips; this soothes the
nervous system.

## OBESITY

If you are obese (weighing 20% or more above the norm) and sleeping badly then your sleep deprivation may reduce the level of growth hormone and this means more of the calories you eat will be converted to . . . fat.

## OVER-SLEEPING

In a book that's all about curing sleeplessness, this really is an oddity. However, many people suffer from it. Over-sleeping will make you feel just about as wretched as sleeplessness; too much sleep leaves the sufferer feeling depressed, lacking in vigilance, full mental ability and co-ordination.

Probable cause: boredom (change jobs and/or find a hobby – see Chapter Two); fear (some underlying problem – see Chapter Seven) or a mental or physical condition for which the over-sleeping is trying, and failing, to compensate (see your health adviser for a check-up and/or lifestyle audit). Probable cure: Read Chapter One again, ie get up at an early, regular time; go to bed later and later to find the right number of sleep hours for you.

## PAIN

Quality sleep does more than give you a "holiday" from your discomfort. It is acknowledged by doctors that the better you sleep the more active the body's healing process. (What is not so well-known is that laughter may be the best pain-killer of all: by stimulating the brain's pleasure centres, the body's own natural pain-killers, the endorphins, are released. They also benefit appetite and sex drive.)

## SLEEPWALKING (Somnambulism or automatism)

Crimes committed whilst sleepwalking will not be punished in law; if sleepwalking is pleaded and cannot be disproved then the "culprit" is considered to have behaved involuntarily, unknowingly and therefore innocently. This dispensation has been granted in the face of some extreme acts; eg, a sleepwalking wife stabbed her husband over a dozen times. She was freed, as was the man (later committed to a mental house) who murdered, then dismembered, his wife whilst he was asleep. Perhaps the most extraordinary case concerned a murder on the beach at a French resort. The detective assigned to the case noticed foot prints around the body; they proved to be his own. The detective himself had shot the victim whilst sleepwalking.

Some sleepwalkers have a penchant for heights and have featured in spectacular and sometimes fatal falls. Cure of the underlying conflict causing the condition will probably be by psychotherapy; meantime, bedroom security is clearly essential.

## SMOKING

Nicotine increases heart rate and blood pressure and is arousing in other ways so smokers will take longer to fall asleep than non-smokers. (Not getting off to sleep causes anxiety, which will make getting off to sleep more difficult, which will cause further anxiety . . .)

## THE WEATHER

Medical opinion in Eastern Europe is firm in the view that we can now blame the weather for some sleep problems: In extremely good weather we need to sleep less; moderate conditions will cause sleep needs to rise and increase further when a weather change is complete. Poor weather has the effect of disturbing our sleep and, not surprisingly, our sleep is liable to be disrupted in extremely unstable conditions.

Well, of course, we knew this all along, didn't we?

Sleep well.

# SECTION FIVE

---

## INFORMATION CHECK LISTS

### CHAPTER 1:   HOW TO GET REGULAR, QUALITY SLEEP
- Eating a mainly cooked diet can lead to tiredness and various other disorders. Read "Raw Energy", by Leslie & Susannah Kenton, pub Century Publishing, £2.25; ISBN 0-7126-0941-4.
- An even more important book is "Food Combining For Health", by Doris Grant and Jean Joice, pub Thorsons, £5.99; ISBN 0-7225-0882-4. A Dr Hay discovered that as the body uses acids to help digest proteins and alkalis to help digest starches, mixing the two in one meal would lead to impaired digestion and possibly even more serious problems.
- "Eat To win" by Dr Robert Haas, pub Viking; ISBN 0-670-80343-X. Haas claims that his diet for winners improves your sex life and the quality of your sleep.
- If stress at work is affecting your sleep then read "Living With Stress" by G. L. Cooper, pub Penguin, £4.95

### CHAPTER 2:   MORE ON HOBBY LISTS & HOW TO USE THEM
- "The Handbook of Chinese Astrology" by Theodora Lau, pub Souvenir Press, £10.95; ISBN 0-285-62725-2.
- "Wallace Milroy's Whisky Almanac", pub Lochar Publishing. £5.95; ISBN 0-948403-12-8.

### A REMINDER LIST OF SOME HOBBIES

| | | |
|---|---|---|
| Aerobics | Ancient monuments | Archaeology |
| Airplanes/models | Angling | Archery |
| Albums | Animals | Architecture |
| American football | Antiques | Arms |
| Amusement machines | Aquaria | Art |

Art needlework
Astrology
Athletics
Autographs
Aviary
Backgammon
Badges
Badminton
Bank notes
Baseball
Basketball
Basket-making
Bee-keeping
Billiards
Bingo
Biology
Boats
Book-binding
Bottles
Boules
Bowling
Boxing
Brass rubbing
Breweriana
Butterflies
Button collecting
CB radio
Cabinet-making
Camping
Candle-making
Canoeing
Classic cars
Caravanning
Card playing
Cardboard cutouts
Carpentry
Carpets
Carving & gilding
Cats
Cattle Breeds
Caving
Ceramics
Charities
Cheese-making
Chess
China & glass
Churchcraft

Cigarette-cards
Clocks & barometers
Cloth-making
Coins & medals
Comics
Computers/games
Concert-going
Confectionery-making
Cookery
Copper-smithing
Costume-making
Crafts
Cricket
Croquet
Cross-country skiing
Cross-words
Curio-collecting
Curling
Cycling & tandems
Dancing
Darts
Design
Detectives
Diving
D-I-Y
Dogs
Dolls
Dominoes
Dowsing
Drama
Draughts
Drawing
Dress-making
Eating out
Embossing
Embroidery
Enamelling
Engraving
Etching
Fancy dress
Fashion designing
Fencing
Flags
Floor painting
Floristry
Flying
Football

Football pools
Fossils
French polishing
Fund raising
Gardening
Genealogy
Geology
Glass blowing
Gliding
Golf
Graphology
Guns
Gymnastics
Hairdressing
Handball
Hang gliding
Heat pump designing
Heraldry
Herbs
Hi-Fi
Hockey
Homoeopathy
Horses
Horticulture
Hunting
Hypnotism
Ice hockey
Ice skating
Illustrating
Insects
Interior decoration
Jewellery
Jigsaws
Jokes
Judo
Juke boxes
Karting
Keep fit
Kilts
Kites
Knitting
Labels
Lace-making
Lacquering
Lacrosse
Landscaping
Languages

Lawn tennis
Leather-work
Lettering
Letter writing
Magic
Mahjong
Maps & charts
Marbling
Martial arts
Metal detecting
Metal restoration
Microlight flying
Microscopy
Military
Mineralogy
Modelling
Monopoly
Motor racing
Mountaineering
Museums
Music
Nature conservation
Naturism
Needlework
Netball
Organ playing
Oriental rugs
Orienteering
Painting
Palmistry
Paper-making
Parachuting
Parliaments
Pavement light-making
Perfume making
Pets
Phonographs
Photography
Photogravure
Picture framing
Pigeons
Play groups/organisers
Plants & Latin names
Polo
Pond-making
Pool playing
Pop stars, hits/charts

Porcelain collecting
Poster-making
Pottery
Poultry breeding
Print making
Printing
Punch & Judy Showman
Puppet making
Putting
Quilting
Radio-controlled models
Railways
Rambling
Recording & taping
Recycling
Reptiles
Rock climbing
Rug making
Rugby football
Saddle making
Scrabble
Script writing (TV/radio)
Scuba diving
Sculpting
Sea-shell collecting
Sewing
Shoe-making
Sight-seeing
Silver-smithing
Skating
Skiing
Skin diving
Snooker
Snorkeling
Social entertaining
Speech-making
Speedway racing
Spinning & weaving
Sports coaching
Squash
Stained glass-making
Stamp collecting
Stencilling
Street light-making
Surfing
Swimming
Table tennis

Taxidermy
Telephones
Textile weaving
Thatching
Theatre
Tickets
Tile designing
Tinbox collecting
Toboganning
Toy making & collecting
Trampolining
Trivial Pursuits
Trophy collecting
Tropical plants growing
T-shirts printing
Typography
TV stars & series
Umbrella collecting
Undertaking
Uniform collecting
Upholstery
Vegetable growing
Video recording
Wallpaper designing
Watch repairs
Water sports
Whisky collecting/
              appreciation
Wig making
Wildlife
Wine making/appreciation
Wire-working
Wood carving
Wool making
Wrestling
Wrought iron design
Yarn marking
Yoga
Zoology

# CHAPTER 3: SOME OPTIONAL AIDS TO GOOD SLEEP

## BEDS
- You get what you pay for. Start by considering Staples' beds; write to them at Windover Rd, Huntingdon, Cambs PE18 7EF, for catalogue. Also look at Swedish producers, Duxiana, 46 George St, London W1H 5RF. If both too expensive then work down through other quality manufacturers until you find the quality/price for you. Remember, if you're going to change, only settle for a quality product.
- Although we may jeer at the idea of a waterbed, situations like not sleeping well and/or aches and pains may be helped by the total body-contouring provided by these. From about £400.
- If money is no problem then the Hypnos Lifestyle slatted bed base may be for you. This super-bed has various tilting systems to adjust head and leg position. Prices according to size and flexibility, but well into four figures!

## THE BEDROOM ITSELF
- "The Natural House Book;" about creating a harmonious, allergy- and bug-free home environment, by D. Pearson, pub Conran Octopus, ISBN 1-85029-175-6.
- Read also, "Interior Design with Feng Shui" by Sarah Rossbach, pub Century, £7.95, ISBN 0-7126-1489-3, for not only how to get the right "Ch'i" in your bedroom but in the rest of your house (and office), too.

## CUDDLES
- Some people are self-conscious about hugging. Read pages 78–82 in "The Art of Sexual Ecstasy" by Margo Anand, pub The Aquarian Press; ISBN 1-85536-007-2.

## FABRICS
- The Cotton Clothing Co, "Cotton On", 29 North Clifton St, Lytham, FY8 5HW, phone 0253 736611. All Swiss-made clothing, no chemical finishes, nylon trimmings or "bad" dyes. For children and adults.

## GURUS and ALTERNATIVE THERAPISTS
A short selection:
- Get details of Ayurveda ("Knowledge of Life", a 5,000–year–old philosophy/therapy) by calling FREEPHONE 0800 269 303. It is claimed that by the use of a wide range of therapies (including meditation, primordial sound, breathing exercise, music and diet, amongst others) cigarette smoking, alcoholism and insomnia, for example, can be cured.
- "Quantum Healing", £5.99, ISBN 0-553-17332-4, and "Perfect Health: The Complete Mind/Body Guide", £7.99, ISBN 0-553-403224-9; both by Dr Deepak Chopra (a qualified doctor and believer/practitioner of Ayurveda), pub Bantam Books. The books tackle in plain language the influence of the mind on bodily function and dysfunction.

- Autogenic Training in Self-Healing: contact Positive Health Centre, 101 Harley St, London W1N 1DF; phone 071 935 1811; for details and addresses of local trainers. AT re-enforces my message that you can head-heal, i.e. mend yourself through your mind.
- Read "Autogenic Training, The Effective Holistic Way To Better Health", by Dr Kai Kermani, pub in hardback by Souvenir Press, £18.50. (Try your local library!)
- Alexander Technique Society of Teachers, 10 London House, 266 Fulham Rd, London SW10; phone 071 351 0828; for teachers of better movement through tuning up neuro-muscular co-ordination. Stored tension can sap energy and adversely affect sleep. Read "The Alexander Principle" by Wilfred Barlow (one of the foremost teachers of the technique), pub Arrow Books; ISBN 0-09-910160-2.
- Yoga: In the round yoga represents a lifestyle rather than a therapy but it is mentioned here because it helps by training the mind to focus *away* from things which are causing it distress and *toward* what can cause pleasure – and sleep. Yoga would not have been with us for so long if it were not beneficial, a view evidently shared by the National Health Service. Try the Stress Research Centre, St Bartholomew's Hospital, Charterhouse Sq, London EC1; phone 071 601 8888. For further information contact Yoga Biomedical Trust, 156 Cockerell Rd, Cambridge; phone 0223 67301, or Yoga for Health Foundation on 0767 27271.
- "Beginner's Guide to Yoga" by N. Phelan, pub Pelham Books, £2.85.
- British Acupuncture Association, 34 Alderney St, London SW1V 4EW; phone 071 834 1012/353. Highly-skilled, practitioners of this needley therapy work by selectively "tapping in" to the body to release trapped, healing energy.
- British Homoeophathic Association, 27a Devonshire St, London W1N 1RJ; phone 071 935 2163. This natural therapy is based on using (often very ancient) remedies prepared from plants and minerals.
- "All In The Mind? Think Yourself Better", by Dr B. Roet, pub MacDonald Optima, £4.95. "Revelations" from the sub-conscious on how we cover up and "rationalise" negative behaviour.
- For a complete run-down on all the alternative therapies available get "The Encyclopedia of Alternative Health Care", by Kristin Olsen, pub in hardback by Piatkus, £15.00. (Library again?).

## HERBS
- Read the herb "bible": "The Herb Book" by John Lust, pub Bantam, £4.95. Everything you could wish to know about herbs and their therapeutic properties. Incidentally, did you know that there are 350 herbal medicine practitioners in the UK? There's bound to be one near you.
- "Harbro" Feather and Down/Herbal Pillows, obtainable from Mrs C. Harding, FREEPOST, "The Maltings Selection", 66 Rembrandt Way, Bury St Edmunds, Suffolk IP33 2LT; phone 0284 752275. £19.95 + p&p.

- The "Breathe-Easy Sinus Pillow". Get it from Health & Beauty Direct, Sutton Fields, Hull HU8 0XD, £16.95 plus p&p £2.

**PILLOWS**
- The sculptured pillow I use is The Pro-Pil-O Neck Support Pillow. This is a German product by Betty Schlafraum-Komfort, Steppdeckerrfabrik Kirchhoff, Postfach 4409, D4400, Munster, but enquire from UK firms selling quality bedding.
- For the smaller person requiring a lower pillow, my wife recommends The Neckcare Pillow, £15.95, from Boots (Code 69-35-745).
- A novel idea for a pillow that may suit you: the "Silver Lining" is a "sandwich" pillow, the "filling" of which is a small, air-inflatable cushion. You blow in the amount of air that produces the ideal pillow bulk for you. Obtainable from Platt & Hill, Belgrave Hill, Keswick Avenue, Oldham, Lancs OL8 2JP; phone 061 626 4628. £24.95 + p&p.

## CHAPTER 4: SLEEPING, DREAMING and SCIENCE: DO THE MYSTERIES LINGER ON?

- "Why We Sleep", by Prof. J. Horne, pub Oxford University Press, £9.95.
- "Sleep and Dreaming", by Dr. Jacob Empson, pub Faber and Faber, £4.99; ISBN 0-571-15181-7.

## CHAPTER 5: PILLS: DRUGGED BODIES ARE PARALYSED, NOT RESTED

- "The Tranquilliser Trap" explains the sleeping pill/tranquilliser problem and gives many valuable addresses where holistic healing is available. Write to The Natural Medicines Society at Edith Lewis House, Back Lane, Ilkeston, Derbys DE7 8EJ; or phone 0602 329454. NMS is a most worthwhile charity fighting to achieve a vital status for the wider use of natural medicines. (They can also use any financial help that you can afford them. Why not consider the very modest subscription and become a member?).
- Track down a recent book, "The Lost Years", by former tranquilliser addict Joan Jerome, for advice on coming off tranquillisers and sleeping pills (she was on 25 a day!); of help to addicts and families.

## CHAPTER 6: SNORING: SOME CAUSES and CURES

- The "Snorestop" Pillow is obtainable for £29.95 from Medipost Ltd, 100 Shaw Rd, Oldham, Lancs OL1 4AY; phone 061 678 0233.
- The "Snore No More" wrist device, ref. no. EP688, £29.95 plus £2.95 p&p, from Innovations (Mail Order) Ltd, Euroway Business Park, Swindon, Wilts SN5 8SN; phone 0792 514666.

- The breathing mask (CPAP) is only one piece of equipment amongst much more hi-tec to be found at 18 sleep centres around the country. Locations are listed in the Appendix on page 59. Do not contact direct; get your doctor to refer you.
- Read "Aromatherapy For Common Ailments", by Shirley Price, pub Gaia Books, £6.99, ISBN 1085675-005-1. Certain essential oils can help soothe and reduce respiratory problems but make sure that you are not allergic to them.

## CHAPTERS 7 & 8: HOW TO FACE & BEAT THE SLEEP-WRECKERS and SLEEP ODDITIES

*Note* Apart from references and help sources for matters raised in the text you will also find below similar information regarding other problems that may be of concern.
Aging; Alcohol; Are Doctors The Only Hope?; Bad Housing; Bereavement (also murder); Children; Debt; Floatation Tank Therapy; Illegal Drug Use; Gambling; Guilt; Job Worries; Laughter; Litigation; Marriage Difficulties; Marriage & Violence; Obesity; Pain; Sick Building Syndrome; Smoking.

### AGING
- Pre-retirement help from Pre-Retirement Association, 0483 39390.
- Age Concern, 081 640 5431 or local phone book for nearest branch.

### ALCOHOL
- Alcoholics Anonymous, PO Box 513, 11 Redcliffe Gardens, London SW10; phone 071 352 3001, for sufferers in London areas; elsewhere, phone 0904 644026.
- Al Anon Family Groups, 61 Gt Dover St, London SE1; phone 071 403 0888 for address of your local group supporting families of those suffering from alcoholism.

### ARE DOCTORS THE ONLY HOPE?
- Read "The Health Crisis", £1.30, from The Natural Medicines Society, Edith Lewis House, Back Lane, Ilkeston, Derbys DE7 8EJ, or phone 0602 329454.

### BAD HOUSING
- Housing Advice Switchboard, 7a/b Fortess Rd, London NW5; phone 071 434 2522.
- For a book on living-in-the-countryside possibilities see DEBT below.

### BEREAVEMENT
- Cruse Bereavement Care, 126 Sheen Rd, Richmond, Surrey TW9 1UR; phone 081 940 4818. Counselling and social contact.

- Compassionate Friends, 6 Denmark St, Bristol BS1 5DQ; phone 0272 292778. Support for bereaved parents. Separate line, 0345 500 800, for families of **murder** victims.

## CHILDREN
- Specialist help: Cry-sis, phone 071 404 5011, for advice on coping with screaming babies. However, before you seek help, research shows that it is normal for babies aged up to three or four months to cry for about two hours in each 24 hours; from this age until about one year old expect the crying to drop to about one hour per 24 hours.
- Check with your local Health Officer to see if there are any special child sleep-problem parent groups in your area.
- Read "Through The Night – Helping Parents & Sleepless Infants" by Dilys Daws, pub Free Association Books, £12.95. Daws is a child psychotherapist who estimates that up to 30% of infants are liable to develop abnormal sleep behaviour, much of which can be traced to underlying family tensions.

## DEBT
- Citizens Financial Advice Bureau, 122 Newgate St, London EC1; phone 071 606 5494.
- There are a number of home-based money-making ideas set out in "Guide To Village Riches", by G. T. Wintour and myself, pub Saturday Richmond Publishers, £5.00; ISBN 1-872804-03-9. Get it from bookshops or direct from SRP, FREEPOST, Haverfordwest, Dyfed SA62 5ZZ, p&p included in price for UK addresses.

## FLOATATION TANK THERAPY
- Send an SAE to The Floatation Tank Assoc, 3A Elms Crescent, London SW4 8QE, for list of locations.

## ILLEGAL DRUG USE
- ISDD (Institute for the Study of Drug Dependence), 1 Hatton Place (off St Cross Street), London EC1N 8ND; phone 071 430 1991. For publications and information.

Self-help groups for drug users are:
- Turning Point, 9-12 Long Lane, London EC1A 9HA; phone 071 606 3947, and
- Narcotics Anonymous, PO Box 417, London SW10 0RS; phone 071 351 6794/6066 (24 hour answerphone).

Self-help organisations for relatives and friends are:
- Adfam National, 82 Old Brompton Rd, London SW7 3LQ; phone 071 823 9313, or
- Families Anonymous, 310 Finchley Rd, London NW3 7AG; phone 071 431 3537, or

- Parentline (Organisations for Parents Under Stress), Rayfa House, 57 Hart Road, Thundersely, Essex SS7 3PD; phone 0268 757077.

## GAMBLING
- Gamblers Anonymous, 17/23 Blantyre St, London SW10; phone 071 352 3060.
- Merseyside Council on Gambling Addictions, 11 Rodney St, Liverpool; phone 051 709 0110.
- They say that "there's always one guy out there who's better than you". Read "13 Against The Bank" by Norman Leigh, pub Oxford University Press, ISBN 0-19-424254-4, in which Leigh tells of his "infallible" system to win at roulette. He did win – but didn't get to keep much money!

## GUILT
- Your local priest is of course a skilled and sympathetic counsellor but if that's too close to home then get the address of your local Samaritans from 0753 32713, or from your local phone book.

## JOB WORRIES
- Vocational Guidance Association, 7 Harley House, Upper Harley St, London NW1; phone 071 935 2600.
- Career Counselling Service, 46 Ferry Rd, London W13; phone 081 741 0335.
- Read "Building A Successful Career or How To Stop Job-Hunting and Start Career-Building", by Alan Jones, pub Business Books, £7.99.
- For an extensive list of alternative occupations see book noted under DEBT.

## LAUGHTER
- Read "Smile Therapy" by Liz Hodgkinson, pub MacDonald Optima; £4.95, ISBN 0-356-12790-7; which tells about the proven, scientific reasons why smiling and laughter are being used as therapy.
- If you want professional endorsement then there's a Dr Dhyan Sutorius who has given up orthodox medicine to run the Centre in Favour of Laughter in Amsterdam!

## LITIGATION
- You can get a free initial consultation with a solicitor who does Legal Aid. Ideally, go to someone who has been recommended; failing that check Yellow Pages for a solicitor near you. No one will ever give you better advice than: "Settle out of court!" The worry, time and unknowable expense makes any court action a lottery.

## MARRIAGE DIFFICULTIES
- To save it: Relate Headquarters, Herbert Gray College, Little Church Street, Rugby CV21 3AP; phone 0788 57324; for a counsellor near you.

- Also, National Family Conciliation Council, 34 Milton St, Swindon SN1 5JA; phone 0793 618486.
- If it's gone, contact National Council for the Divorced and Separated, 13 High St, Little Shelford, Cambridge CB2 5ES; phone 021 588 5757 (they have over 100 branches in the UK); or Divorce Conciliation & Advisory Service on 071 730 2422.
- And read "Splitting Up: A Legal and Financial Guide to Separation and Divorce", by David Green, pub Kogan Page; ISBN 1-850917663, £5.95. Green is a solicitor and an expert on family law (and has been divorced!).

## MARRIAGE AND VIOLENCE
- Should this be part of the problem in the home then immediately contact Lifeline on 0793 73286 for the phone number of your local group.

## OBESITY
- Read "Food Facts" by Carol Rinzler, pub Bloomsbury Publishing and "Complete Nutrition" by Michael Sharon, pub Prion.
- Read "Food Combining For Health – A New Look at the Hay System" by Doris Grant & Jean Joice, Thorsons, ISBN 0-7225-0882-4.
- Over-eaters Anonymous, Pinner, Middx; phone 081 868 4109, or London 081 981 9363.
- Weight Watchers (UK) Ltd, 11 Fairacres, Dedworth Rd, Windsor; phone 071 580 4765, for the address of a local branch; but if it's really making you feel desperate then contact
- The Samaritans, phone 0753 32713, or check your local directory for a help line near you.

## PAIN
- Many self-help groups, so get specific advice from The Medical Advisory Service, phone 081 994 6477; or Patients Association, 0703 779091 or 0703 777222 ext 3753.
- Read "Anatomy Of An Illness" by Norman Cousins, pub Bantam, £3.95; ISBN 0-553-17363-4. Cousins was "terminally" ill but couldn't accept the prognosis and wouldn't lie down and die. He used laughter as therapy and survived!
- Read "The Fantasy Factor" by Dr H E Stanton, pub MacDonald Optima, £3.95, which suggests ways of using the imagination to overcome pain and negative thinking.

## SICK BUILDING SYNDROME
- Certain buildings and the things in them can cause illness, allergies and sleeplessness. For fuller information on polluting materials read "The Natural House Book" by D. Reason, pub Conran Octopus; ISBN 1-85029-175-6.
- According to NASA, some plants will zap the harmful effects of certain pollutants, eg, carbon monoxide and formaldehyde (from synthetic carpets and some furniture) will be removed from the air by Spider Plants;

benzine (a cancer-causer from cleaning fluids) will be absorbed by Ivy, Gerbera Daisy or Chrysanthemum; computer screen emissions can be countered by the cactus Cereus Peruvianus.

- For a special package of house/office-friendly plant seeds that will also tackle the pollution of cigarette smoke, hairsprays, deodrants, fly spray, shoe polish, photocopier and computer emissions etc get an Amway Environment Kit. Contact Amway UK Ltd, Snowdon Drive, Winterhill, Milton Keynes, MK6 1AR; phone 0908 679888.

## SMOKING

- Smokers Information & Advice Centre (QUIT), 40 Hanson St, London W1; phone 071 636 9103, for help in tracking down a group near you. Or ASH (Action on Smoking & Health) on 071 637 9843.
- Also read "Kick It!" by Judy Perlmutter, pub Thorsons, £2.99; ISBN 0-7225-1523-5. She claims an 80% success rate.
- If snuffing not smoking could help then contact G. Smith & Sons, 74 Charing Cross Rd, London WC2H; phone 071 836 7422 for their snuff catalogue and advice.

# BIBLIOGRAPHY

The Body Machine, ed Christian Barnard
Raw Energy, L & S Kenton
Food Combining For Health – A New Look at the Hay System, D Grant &
J Joice
Eat To Win, Dr R Haas
Living With Stress, G L Cooper
Handbook of Chinese Astrology, T Lau
Wallace Milroy's Whisky Almanac, W Milroy
The Natural House Book, D Pearson
Interior Design With Feng Shui, S Rossbach
The Art of Sexual Ecstasy, M Anand
Quantum Healing, Dr D Chopra
Perfect Health: The Complete Mind/Body Guide, Dr D Chopra
Autogenic Training, The Effective Holistic Way To Better Health, Dr K
Kermani
The Alexander Principle, W Barlow
Beginner's Guide To Yoga, N Phelan
All In The Mind? Think Yourself Better, Dr R Roet
The Encyclopedia of Alternative Health Care, K Olsen
The Herb Book, J Lust
Why We Sleep, Prof J Horne
Sleep & Dreaming, Dr J Empson
The Tranquilliser Trap, pub Natural Medicines Society
The Lost Years, J Jerome
Aromatherapy for Common Ailments, S Price
The Health Crisis, pub Natural Medicines Society
Through The Night – Helping Parents & Sleepless Infants, D Daws
13 Against The Bank, N Leigh
Building A Successful Career/How To Stop Job-Hunting & Start Career-
Building, A Jones
Smile Therapy, L Hodgkinson
Splitting Up: A Legal & Financial Guide to Separation & Divorce, D Green
Food Facts, C Rinzler
Complete Nutrition, M Sharon
Anatomy of An Illness, N Cousins
The Fantasy Factor, Dr H E Stanton
Kick It!, J Perlmutter
Wimbledon Men, The Singles Champions, A Little and L Tingay

# INDEX

# APPENDIX: Specialist Sleep Units

By getting your doctor to refer you to one of the doctors in charge of the appropriate unit near you, you can be sure that whatever your problem (particularly if it is stubborn snoring) this will be professionally analysed and a cure prescribed.

## LONDON
Dr P J Rees
Guy's Hospital, SE1

Dr J Wedzicha
London Chest Hospital, E2

Mr C B Croft
Royal National Ear
Nose & Throat Hospital, WC1

Prof A Guz
Charing Cross Hospital, W6

Dr K Simonds
Royal Brompton National
Heart and Lung Hospital, SW3

## ENGLAND
Dr P Meisner
Breakspear Hospital,
Abbots Langley, Herts WD5

Dr J R Stradling
Churchill Hospital
Oxford, Oxon OX3

Dr J R Catterall
Bristol Royal Infirmary
Bristol, BS2

Dr A Ferguson
Wonford House Hospital
Exeter, Devon

Dr T J Coady
Ipswich Hospital
Ipswich, Suffolk

Dr J M Shneerson
Newmarket General Hospital
Newmarket, Suffolk

Dr C D Hanning
Leicester General Hospital
Leicester LE5

Dr K Prowse
City General Hospital
Stoke on Trent, Staffs ST4

Dr P Howard
Royal Hallamshire Hospital
Sheffield

Dr A Woodcock
Wythenshawe Hospital
Manchester M23

Dr P M Calverley
Fazakerley Hospital
Fazakerley, Liverpool L9

## WALES
Dr A P Smith
Llandough Hospital
Penarth, South Glam CF6

## SCOTLAND
Dr N J Douglas
City Hospital, Edinburgh EH10

## NORTHERN IRELAND
Dr I Gleadhill
Belfast City Hospital

Also from Saturday Richmond Publishers

## GUIDE TO VILLAGE RICHES

### by G. T. Wintour & Zachariah Evans

- Surveys show that most of us would really prefer to live in the space and health of a countryside home; with the growing trend to home-working the time's right to acquire and reinvent a country home and make your money and a career there as well.
- Written by people who have made the switch from city to village home/workbase GUIDE TO VILLAGE RICHES tells you all you need to know to turn this dream into reality, eg:
- Don't buy your country home ○ Save your money for one of the 36 fulfilling country businesses outlined ○ Some businesses (and "experts") to treat with caution ○ Keep your job whilst you start a venture ○ Children's education ○ Finding new country friends ○ How to pick a venture for your personality and profit ○ Street-wise borrowing ○ Getting the best price for your present home ○ Training and retraining ○ GUIDE TO VILLAGE RICHES will get you where you want to be – COUNTRYSIDE!

**What the reviewers said. . .**

"Novel. Useful compendium of tips, ideas and information for those tired of city life but nervous of economic survival in the countryside . . . valuable."
**– THE INDEPENDENT ON SUNDAY**

"More than 360 pages bursting with ideas from the ordinary to the extraordinary. . ." **– BBC RADIO**

"The Guide is crammed with hints, facts, names and addresses . . . stimulating."
**– FARM DEVELOPMENT REVIEW**

"It offers 36 money-spinning ideas. . ." **– TODAY**

As a very welcome new Saturday Richmond customer we are pleased to offer you GUIDE TO VILLAGE RICHES at the **DISCOUNT PRICE** of £5.00, to include p&p (UK only). Non-UK residents please add £3.00 to cover insurance, airmail postage & packaging to price. Sterling cheques, please.

Orders to:

SATURDAY RICHMOND PUBLISHERS
FREEPOST
BS7663, Pilning, Bristol, BS12 3BR